AYEMOBA BRAIMAH

# The Well-Balanced Pharmacist: Reducing Work-Related Stress in Pharmacy Practice

First edition

This book was professionally typeset on Reedsy.
Find out more at reedsy.com

# Contents

# 1

# Chapter 1: Understanding the Stress in Pharmacy Practice

P harmacy practice is an integral part of healthcare, making significant contributions to patient health and wellbeing. Pharmacists bear the tremendous responsibility of ensuring medications are safely and accurately dispensed. But this critical role is not without its challenges. Pharmacists often face high levels of job-related stress stemming from various factors. By understanding these stressors, pharmacists can better identify and manage them to maintain a healthy and fulfilling career.

**High Demand**

One of the most common stressors in pharmacy practice is the high demand for services. With the aging population and increased prevalence of chronic diseases, the demand for medications and pharmaceutical care is continually rising. Pharmacists may find themselves handling more prescriptions than ever before, which can increase the pressure to work quickly and efficiently. Moreover, pharmacists are expected to provide a wider range of services beyond dispensing medications, such as administering vaccines, conducting health screenings, and providing medication therapy management.

**Rigorous Protocols**

Pharmacy practice involves strict adherence to protocols and guidelines to ensure patient safety. Pharmacists must meticulously follow these protocols when dispensing medications, checking doses, assessing potential drug interactions, and providing patient counseling. The high stakes nature of these tasks, where a mistake could lead to severe health consequences for a patient, can contribute to a significant amount of stress.

### Attention to Detail

Attention to detail is paramount in pharmacy practice. Pharmacists must ensure the right medication at the right dose is given to the right patient. They need to check and double-check every prescription, which can be time-consuming and mentally exhausting, particularly during busy periods. This need for precision, while necessary, can add to the pressure and stress experienced by pharmacists.

### Multitasking

Pharmacists often have to juggle multiple tasks at once. They may be dispensing medications, counseling patients, answering phone calls, and dealing with administrative tasks, all at the same time. This constant multitasking can lead to cognitive overload, contributing to fatigue and stress.

### Patient Interactions

While interacting with patients can be rewarding, it can also be stressful. Pharmacists may encounter challenging situations, such as dealing with difficult or demanding patients, explaining complex medication regimens, or delivering bad news. These emotionally charged interactions can be a significant source of stress.

### Long Hours and Shift Work

Many pharmacists work long hours, including evenings, nights, and weekends. The irregular and extended working hours can disrupt sleep patterns, lead to fatigue, and impact work-life balance, all of which can contribute to stress.

### Professional Isolation

In some settings, pharmacists may work alone or with limited interaction with other healthcare professionals. This professional isolation can be stressful, as pharmacists may feel unsupported and overwhelmed by the responsibility they bear.

This chapter serves as an introduction to the various stressors faced by pharmacists in their practice. The subsequent chapters will delve deeper into each of these stressors and provide strategies to manage and reduce stress effectively.

# 2

# Chapter 2: Identifying Sources of Stress

I dentifying your unique sources of stress is the first step in formulating an effective stress management plan. Stress in the pharmacy workplace can be influenced by several factors. These factors could be personal, related to your work environment, or linked to the broader healthcare system. Understanding these potential stressors can help you to anticipate, prepare for, and manage stress more effectively. This chapter will guide you through the process of identifying your unique sources of stress in your pharmacy practice.

**Personal Stressors**

Individual personality traits and personal circumstances can significantly influence how you perceive and respond to stress. Some individuals may thrive in a fast-paced environment, while others may find it overwhelming. To identify personal stressors:

1. **Self-Reflection:** Take time to reflect on how you react to stress. Do you tend to get anxious easily? Do you find it hard to let go of mistakes? Knowing your tendencies can help you recognize when you are feeling stressed and identify what triggers these feelings.
2. **Work-Life Balance:** Evaluate your work-life balance. Are you finding it difficult to switch off from work during your downtime? Are your work commitments interfering with your personal life or family time?

Identifying such imbalances can reveal a significant source of stress.

## Work Environment Stressors

Your work environment can contribute significantly to your stress levels. Some potential stressors include:

1. **Workload:** A heavy workload, with a high volume of prescriptions to fill and patients to counsel, can lead to stress. Monitor your workload and note periods when you feel overwhelmed.
2. **Interpersonal Relationships:** Interactions with colleagues and patients can sometimes be challenging. Pay attention to any situations or individuals that regularly cause you stress.
3. **Lack of Control:** Feeling like you have little control over your work can be a major stressor. This might be due to inflexible work hours, inadequate input into decision-making, or lack of autonomy in your role.
4. **Lack of Support:** A lack of support from management or colleagues can exacerbate stress. If you feel unsupported or undervalued in your role, it's essential to recognize this as a potential source of stress.

## System-Level Stressors

System-level factors can also contribute to workplace stress. These can include:

1. **Regulatory Demands:** Keeping up with evolving regulations and guidelines can be stressful. If you are finding it hard to stay updated or implement changes, this could be a significant source of stress.
2. **Technological Challenges:** Technology can make tasks more efficient, but it can also be a source of stress if systems are complex, unreliable, or frequently changing.
3. **Organizational Change:** Changes in the organization's structure or strategies can cause uncertainty and stress. Noticing your reactions to these changes can help you identify this as a stressor.

To help identify these sources of stress, consider keeping a stress journal. Document instances when you feel stressed, noting what you were doing, who you were interacting with, and any deadlines or demands you were facing. Over time, you will likely see patterns emerge, and you can use these insights to develop strategies to manage these stressors effectively.

In the next chapters, we will explore how to manage these identified sources of stress and create a more balanced and less stressful pharmacy practice.

# 3

# Chapter 3: The Art of Delegation

E ffective delegation is an essential skill for managing stress in the pharmacy practice. By sharing responsibilities, you can balance workloads, free up time for essential tasks, and create a collaborative and supportive work environment. Delegation is an art that requires trust, clear communication, and understanding of your team's capabilities. This chapter will guide you on how to delegate effectively in your pharmacy practice.

**Recognize the Need for Delegation**

Pharmacists often feel the need to handle every task due to the sensitive nature of their work. However, managing all tasks alone can lead to a heavy workload and increased stress. Recognize that delegation is not about passing off work—it's about efficiently managing resources and promoting teamwork.

**Understand Your Team**

To delegate effectively, you need to understand your team's strengths, weaknesses, and interests. Spend time observing their work, offer regular feedback, and have open conversations about their aspirations and areas for development. This understanding can help you assign tasks that align with their skills and career goals, leading to better job satisfaction and performance.

**Prioritize Tasks**

Not all tasks need your direct attention. The Eisenhower Matrix is a useful tool for prioritizing tasks. It categorizes tasks into four quadrants:

1. **Urgent and important (tasks you will do immediately).**
2. **Important, but not urgent (tasks you will schedule to do later).**
3. **Urgent, but not important (tasks you will delegate).**
4. **Neither urgent nor important (tasks that you will eliminate).**

By categorizing tasks, you can identify what tasks you need to handle yourself and what can be safely delegated.

### Clearly Define Tasks and Expectations

Once you've decided which tasks to delegate, clearly define the task, expectations, and desired outcomes. Ensure the person understands what is expected, the task's importance, and how it fits into the larger picture. Clarify any doubts and reassure them that you are available for any questions or help.

### Empower and Trust Your Team

Delegation involves entrusting others to complete tasks. Allow your team to take ownership, make decisions, and learn from their mistakes. This trust can motivate your team, increase their confidence, and enhance their skills.

### Provide Resources and Support

Ensure your team has the necessary resources to complete the tasks. This includes access to information, tools, and time. Provide support and guidance when needed but avoid micromanaging.

### Monitor Progress and Provide Feedback

Keep track of the progress without interfering in the process. Offer constructive feedback to help your team improve. Appreciate their efforts and acknowledge their contributions. This recognition can boost morale and encourage them to take on more responsibilities.

Delegation can significantly reduce your workload and stress. It requires practice and patience, but over time it can lead to a more balanced and effective pharmacy practice.

# 4

# Chapter 4: Efficient Workflow Management

E fficient workflow management is pivotal in reducing stress within the pharmacy environment. It can increase productivity, streamline processes, reduce errors, and promote a more balanced and less hectic work environment. Implementing efficient workflows requires planning, organization, and regular evaluation for improvements. This chapter will guide you through steps to effectively manage your pharmacy workflow.

**Assess the Current Workflow**

The first step is to assess your current workflow. Observe the processes, identify bottlenecks, and note any tasks or steps that seem redundant or inefficient. Pay attention to any processes that cause frustration or delays, as these may be areas where improvements can be made.

**Map Your Processes**

Create a visual map of your workflow, starting from receiving the prescription to dispensing the medication to the patient. Mapping your process can help you visualize the sequence of tasks, identify dependencies, and pinpoint areas of inefficiency.

**Prioritize and Organize Tasks**

Not all tasks are equally important. Prioritize tasks based on urgency and importance. Use tools such as the Eisenhower Matrix, discussed in the previous chapter, to help with prioritization. Organize tasks in a way that reduces back-and-forth movement, minimizes interruptions, and allows for smooth transitions from one task to another.

### Implement Technology

Technology can greatly enhance workflow efficiency. Electronic health records (EHRs), pharmacy management systems, and automated dispensing machines can streamline processes, reduce manual tasks, and minimize errors. Implement technology where feasible and train your staff adequately to use it effectively.

### Delegate Responsibilities

Assign tasks based on your team's skills, strengths, and licensure. As discussed in the previous chapter, effective delegation can balance workloads, promote teamwork, and reduce stress. Ensure everyone knows their responsibilities and how their work fits into the overall workflow.

### Maintain a Clean and Organized Workspace

An organized workspace can improve efficiency and reduce errors. Arrange supplies logically and maintain a clean and clutter-free workspace. This includes digital organization—clearly label digital files and use folders to keep your computer organized.

### Standardize Processes

Standardization can reduce confusion, enhance efficiency, and ensure consistency in quality. Create standard operating procedures (SOPs) for common tasks and ensure all staff are trained on these procedures.

### Continuous Improvement

Workflow management is not a one-time task. Regularly review your workflow, invite feedback from your team, and be open to making adjustments. Continuous improvement can help you adapt to changes and maintain an efficient workflow.

Efficient workflow management can create a smoother, less stressful pharmacy practice. It may take time to implement and adjust to new workflows, but the resulting improvements in productivity and reductions in stress will be well worth the effort.

5

# Chapter 5: Integrating Automation in Pharmacy

Automation has revolutionized various aspects of healthcare, and pharmacy is no exception. Automation, when appropriately integrated, can reduce repetitive tasks, minimize errors, improve efficiency, and ultimately reduce stress in the pharmacy practice. This chapter provides an overview of how to effectively leverage automation in your pharmacy.

**Types of Automation in Pharmacy**

There are several types of automation that can be useful in a pharmacy setting:

1. **Automated Dispensing Cabinets (ADCs):** ADCs dispense medications at the push of a button, reducing the time spent on manual dispensing and minimizing errors.
2. **Robot-Assisted Dispensing Systems:** These are used in larger pharmacies and hospitals. They can accurately dispense and package high volumes of medication, saving time and reducing strain on pharmacists.
3. **Pharmacy Management Systems:** These systems automate administrative tasks such as inventory management, billing, and reporting, reducing the burden of paperwork and manual record-keeping.

4. **E-prescribing:** E-prescribing enables physicians to send prescriptions directly to the pharmacy, reducing wait times and transcription errors.

5. **Automated Compounding Systems:** These systems accurately measure and mix ingredients for compounded prescriptions, ensuring precision and consistency.

## Benefits of Automation

Automation offers several benefits that can reduce stress in pharmacy practice:

1. **Efficiency:** Automation can greatly speed up repetitive tasks, freeing up time for pharmacists to focus on more critical responsibilities such as patient counseling and clinical services.

2. **Reduced Errors:** Automated systems can reduce human errors in dispensing and compounding medications, ensuring patient safety and reducing the stress associated with potential mistakes.

3. **Improved Workflow:** Automation can streamline workflow, reduce bottlenecks, and create a smoother, less stressful work environment.

4. **Data Analysis:** Automated systems can generate reports and analytics that can help you make data-driven decisions, improve operations, and manage inventory more efficiently.

## Integrating Automation

While automation can provide significant benefits, it must be integrated thoughtfully to ensure a positive impact. Here are some steps to consider:

1. **Identify Needs:** Evaluate your current workflow and identify tasks that could be automated. These might include time-consuming, repetitive tasks, or tasks prone to error.

2. **Research Options:** Once you've identified tasks that could benefit from automation, research the different automation options available. Consider factors like cost, space, ease of use, and integration with your existing systems.

3. **Training:** When introducing new technology, ensure adequate training for all staff. This includes not just how to use the technology, but also understanding its benefits and limitations.

4. **Monitor and Evaluate:** After implementing automation, regularly monitor and evaluate its impact. Make adjustments as needed to ensure it's contributing positively to your workflow and reducing stress.

Automation can transform your pharmacy practice, reducing stress, and improving efficiency. As technology continues to advance, even more opportunities for automation will likely emerge, making it an area to watch in the coming years.

6

# Chapter 6: Communication and Interpersonal Relationships

E ffective communication is foundational in any professional setting, and pharmacy is no exception. It can reduce misunderstandings, resolve conflicts, and foster a supportive work environment, all of which can significantly alleviate work-related stress. Additionally, it enhances patient care by ensuring clear and concise conveyance of health information. This chapter delves into how effective communication and healthy interpersonal relationships can mitigate stress in pharmacy practice.

**The Power of Effective Communication**

Communication is a two-way process: it involves both conveying your own thoughts and understanding others'. Here are some strategies to enhance communication:

1. **Clarity:** Be clear and concise in your communication to avoid confusion and misunderstanding. This is particularly important when discussing medication instructions with patients.
2. **Active Listening:** Active listening involves fully focusing on the speaker, showing empathy, and providing feedback. This can lead to better understanding and collaboration with colleagues and patients.
3. **Non-verbal Communication:** Be mindful of your body language, tone

of voice, and facial expressions, as these can convey a lot of information beyond your words.

4. **Open Dialogue:** Encourage an open dialogue where everyone feels comfortable expressing their thoughts and concerns. This can foster a supportive work environment and improve problem-solving.

## Building Healthy Interpersonal Relationships

Healthy relationships with colleagues and patients can greatly reduce work stress. Here's how you can nurture these relationships:

1. **Respect:** Treat everyone with kindness and respect. This can foster a positive work environment and build strong, trusting relationships.
2. **Teamwork:** Encourage a sense of teamwork where everyone's contributions are valued and recognized. This can lead to better collaboration and reduce feelings of isolation.
3. **Conflict Resolution:** Address conflicts promptly and constructively. Unresolved conflicts can escalate and cause significant stress. Use conflicts as an opportunity to improve relationships and find solutions.
4. **Patient Interaction:** Building strong relationships with patients can be rewarding and reduce stress. Show empathy, provide patient-centered care, and take time to understand their needs.

## Communication with Patients

In a pharmacy setting, communication with patients is crucial. Here are some tips to improve this communication:

1. **Patient Counseling:** Be patient and empathetic when counseling patients. Use layman's terms to explain medication instructions and side effects.
2. **Privacy:** Respect patient privacy. Hold sensitive conversations in a private area to make patients feel more comfortable.
3. **Follow-up:** Follow-up with patients to ensure they are taking their medications correctly. This not only improves patient outcomes but also builds trust and rapport.

Effective communication and healthy interpersonal relationships can greatly reduce work stress and improve job satisfaction. These skills might take time to develop, but they are well worth the effort and can significantly improve your pharmacy practice.

# 7

# Chapter 7: Developing Emotional Resilience

Emotional resilience refers to one's ability to adapt to stressful situations or crises. In the high-stakes, high-stress world of pharmacy, emotional resilience is vital. It can help pharmacists handle daily pressures, bounce back from adversity, and reduce the likelihood of burnout. This chapter offers practical advice on building emotional resilience.

**Understanding Emotional Resilience**

Emotional resilience is not about avoiding stress or hardships but rather learning how to manage and adapt to them. It involves being able to "bounce back" from difficult experiences and maintaining a positive outlook.

**Key Components of Emotional Resilience**

1. **Self-Awareness:** Recognize your emotions and understand why you feel a certain way. Self-awareness is the first step towards managing your emotions effectively.
2. **Self-Regulation:** Learn to manage your reactions to stress and avoid impulsive behaviors. This can involve techniques like deep breathing, meditation, or taking a step back from a situation before responding.
3. **Mental Agility:** Try to view challenges from different perspectives. By shifting your mindset, you can find better ways to cope with stress and solve problems.

4. **Optimism:** Maintain a hopeful outlook. While it's important to be realistic, optimism can help you stay motivated and focused on solutions.

5. **Self-Care:** Regular physical exercise, balanced nutrition, adequate sleep, and relaxation are essential for emotional resilience.

## Building Emotional Resilience

Here are some practical strategies to build emotional resilience:

1. **Develop Stress Management Techniques:** Techniques such as deep breathing, yoga, meditation, and progressive muscle relaxation can reduce stress levels and enhance your ability to manage difficult situations.

2. **Cultivate Positive Relationships:** Build strong, supportive relationships both in and outside work. Social support can provide a sense of belonging and help you navigate through tough times.

3. **Practice Mindfulness:** Mindfulness involves staying present and fully engaged in the current moment. It can reduce anxiety, improve mood, and help you respond to stress more effectively.

4. **Stay Physically Active:** Regular physical activity can reduce stress, improve mood, and boost your energy levels. Find an activity you enjoy and make it a part of your routine.

5. **Seek Professional Help:** If stress becomes overwhelming, seek help from a mental health professional. Therapy can provide tools and strategies to manage stress and build emotional resilience.

Building emotional resilience can be a journey, but it's one that can lead to greater well-being, reduced stress, and a more fulfilling pharmacy practice. Remember, it's okay to ask for help and take time for yourself. After all, taking care of your mental health is a key part of being able to provide the best care for your patients.

# 8

# Chapter 8: Prioritizing Mental Health

**M**ental health plays an integral role in our overall wellbeing and our ability to cope with stress. For pharmacists, prioritizing mental health can lead to better job performance, increased job satisfaction, and improved relationships with colleagues and patients. This chapter delves into why mental health is crucial in managing work-related stress and provides strategies to incorporate mindfulness and other self-care practices into your daily routine.

**Understanding the Role of Mental Health**

Mental health is more than the absence of mental disorders; it's a state of well-being in which individuals realize their abilities, can cope with normal life stresses, can work productively, and contribute to their community. Here are some reasons why mental health should be prioritized:

1. **Performance and Productivity:** Poor mental health can lead to decreased concentration, decision-making skills, and productivity—all vital aspects of a pharmacist's role.

2. **Workplace Relationships:** Mental wellbeing can influence how we interact with others. By maintaining good mental health, pharmacists can build better relationships with colleagues and patients.

3. **Job Satisfaction:** Prioritizing mental health can lead to higher job satisfaction. Enjoying what you do and finding purpose in your work

can contribute to a healthier, happier mindset.

4. **Resilience:** Good mental health enhances resilience, allowing pharmacists to better handle daily pressures and bounce back from adversity.

## Strategies to Prioritize Mental Health

1. **Mindfulness:** Mindfulness involves focusing on the present moment without judgment. Regular mindfulness practice can reduce stress, improve focus, and enhance emotional wellbeing. Incorporate mindfulness into your daily routine—perhaps during a morning meditation, on a lunchtime walk, or while preparing for bed.

2. **Self-care:** Self-care involves activities that you enjoy and that contribute to your wellbeing. This might be reading, exercising, spending time in nature, cooking a healthy meal, or spending time with loved ones. Ensure you make time for self-care activities daily.

3. **Mental Health Days:** If possible, taking mental health days when you feel overwhelmed can help recharge your mental batteries. These are just as important as taking time off for physical illness.

4. **Professional Help:** If you're feeling consistently overwhelmed, anxious, or low, seek help from a mental health professional. They can provide strategies to manage stress and improve mental wellbeing.

5. **Healthy Lifestyle:** A balanced diet, regular physical activity, adequate sleep, and avoiding harmful levels of substance use all contribute to better mental health.

6. **Social Connections:** Maintain strong relationships with colleagues, friends, and family. Social support can provide a sense of belonging and help you navigate through tough times.

By making mental health a priority, pharmacists can better manage stress and enhance their quality of life. Remember, it's okay to ask for help and take time for yourself. After all, your mental health matters—for your own wellbeing and for the quality of care you provide to your patients.

# 9

# Chapter 9: Physical Well-Being and Stress

P hysical health plays a significant role in managing stress. By maintaining our physical well-being, we can better cope with stressors and improve our overall health and vitality. In addition, certain physical habits can significantly impact our mood, energy levels, and ability to think clearly—all critical factors in the demanding field of pharmacy. This chapter explores the connection between physical health and stress and provides tips on nutrition, exercise, and adequate rest.

### The Physical Health-Stress Connection

There's a powerful connection between our physical health and stress. When we're stressed, our bodies release hormones like cortisol and adrenaline that prepare us for a "fight or flight" response. While these hormones can be helpful in short-term, high-stress situations, they can be harmful when their levels remain high for prolonged periods—something that can occur due to chronic stress.

Over time, chronic stress can contribute to a range of physical health issues, including heart disease, diabetes, gastrointestinal problems, and weakened immune function. On the flip side, when we take care of our physical health—through good nutrition, regular exercise, and adequate rest—we can enhance our body's ability to manage stress.

### Nutrition

Eating a healthy, balanced diet can help you cope with stress by stabilizing your energy levels and mood. Here are some nutritional tips:

1. **Eat Regular, Balanced Meals:** Regular meals can prevent energy slumps during the day. Include a balance of complex carbohydrates, lean proteins, and healthy fats in your meals.
2. **Stay Hydrated:** Dehydration can lead to fatigue and difficulty concentrating. Aim to drink at least eight glasses of water a day, more if you're physically active or it's a hot day.
3. **Limit Caffeine and Alcohol:** While these substances might seem to help with stress in the short term, they can lead to increased anxiety and sleep issues over time.
4. **Eat Plenty of Fruits and Vegetables:** They're packed with vitamins, minerals, and fiber that can boost your immune system and overall health.

**Exercise**

Physical activity can be an effective stress reliever. Here's why:

1. **Endorphin Release:** Exercise triggers the release of endorphins—your body's natural mood lifters.
2. **Improved Sleep:** Regular physical activity can help you sleep better, which can improve your mood and energy levels.
3. **Distraction:** Exercise can provide a break from stressors, giving your mind a chance to rest and refocus.

Try to incorporate at least 30 minutes of moderate-intensity exercise—such as brisk walking, cycling, or swimming—into your daily routine.

**Rest**

Adequate rest is essential for managing stress. Lack of sleep can affect your mood, energy levels, and ability to handle stress. Try to get 7-9 hours of sleep per night. Develop a regular sleep schedule and create a restful environment to promote better sleep.

By prioritizing your physical health, you'll not only feel better physically but also be better equipped to handle stress. Remember, managing stress is not just about dealing with mental and emotional challenges—it's about taking care of your whole self, body included.

# 10

# Chapter 10: Managing External Pressures

While pharmacy work undoubtedly has its share of stresses, we cannot overlook the fact that external pressures also contribute significantly to overall stress levels. Familial responsibilities, financial stressors, and even societal pressures can pile onto the stress experienced at work, leading to a sense of overwhelm. This chapter provides strategies to manage these external pressures to help reduce overall stress levels and maintain a healthier work-life balance.

**Understanding External Pressures**

External pressures often stem from areas of our lives outside work. They may include responsibilities towards family and loved ones, financial obligations and worries, societal expectations, or even personal health issues. While these pressures may not be directly related to your job as a pharmacist, they can affect your stress levels, job performance, and overall wellbeing.

**Managing Family and Personal Responsibilities**

Balancing work responsibilities with family and personal life can be challenging. Here are some strategies to manage these responsibilities:

1. **Set Boundaries:** Make it clear to your family when you're working and when you can spend time with them. Use this same principle to define your personal time.
2. **Shared Responsibilities:** Share household chores and responsibilities

with family members to avoid taking on too much yourself.

3. **Quality Time:** Ensure you spend quality time with your loved ones. While it's about quantity, quality matters. Plan activities that everyone enjoys.

4. **Seek Help:** If needed, seek help from professional services such as childcare, eldercare, or home maintenance services to reduce your load.

## Managing Financial Stress

Financial stress can be a significant source of anxiety. Here's how to manage it:

1. **Budgeting:** Create a budget to keep track of income and expenses. This can help avoid overspending and ensure you live within your means.

2. **Savings and Investments:** Try to save a portion of your income regularly. Invest wisely for future needs and to create an emergency fund.

3. **Debt Management:** If you're in debt, create a plan to pay it off. Seek advice from a financial advisor if necessary.

4. **Insurance:** Ensure you have appropriate insurance coverage—like health, life, and property—to manage unexpected expenses.

## Dealing with Societal Pressures

Societal pressures can come from expectations about lifestyle, appearance, or status. Here are ways to manage these pressures:

1. **Self-Acceptance:** Accept yourself as you are. Remember that everyone is unique and that there's no one-size-fits-all in life.

2. **Positive Social Circle:** Surround yourself with positive people who respect and support you.

3. **Limit Social Media:** Excessive social media use can increase feelings of inadequacy and stress. Limit your use and remember that people often only post their highlights—not their everyday reality.

Remember, managing external pressures is about finding a balance that works for you. While it's essential to fulfill your responsibilities, it's equally important to care for your health and wellbeing. After all, being the best pharmacist you can be means taking care of yourself both at work and outside of it.

# 11

# Chapter 11: Strengthening Coping Mechanisms

C oping mechanisms are strategies that individuals use to manage stress and navigate through challenging situations. They can greatly influence how we react to stress, making the difference between healthy stress management and the potential onset of burnout. This chapter is dedicated to identifying and developing strong coping mechanisms that can help you handle high-stress situations effectively.

**Understanding Coping Mechanisms**

Coping mechanisms can be divided into two primary types: adaptive (or healthy) coping strategies, which promote stress management and well-being, and maladaptive (or unhealthy) coping strategies, which may provide temporary relief but can cause long-term harm.

Examples of adaptive coping mechanisms include problem-solving, seeking social support, exercising, practicing mindfulness, and using relaxation techniques. Maladaptive coping mechanisms may include excessive alcohol consumption, procrastination, overeating, or excessive sleeping.

It's important to recognize that while maladaptive strategies might offer immediate relief, they can exacerbate stress levels in the long run. On the other hand, adaptive strategies may require more effort upfront but lead to more effective stress management over time.

**Developing Strong Coping Mechanisms**

1. **Identify Existing Mechanisms:** The first step is to identify the coping mechanisms you currently use. You may already employ some adaptive strategies without realizing it. Recognizing these strategies can help reinforce their use.

2. **Explore New Strategies:** If you feel your current coping strategies aren't sufficient, consider exploring new ones. Research different techniques, speak to a mental health professional, or talk to peers about what they find effective.

3. **Practicing Mindfulness:** Mindfulness can help you stay centered in high-stress situations. By focusing on the present, you can prevent stress about the past or future from overwhelming you.

4. **Physical Activity:** Exercise is a great way to relieve stress and clear your mind. It doesn't have to be high-intensity—a brisk walk can be just as beneficial.

5. **Seeking Social Support:** Reaching out to others for support can significantly help manage stress. This could be friends, family, a mentor, or a support group of peers experiencing similar challenges.

6. **Relaxation Techniques:** Techniques such as deep breathing, progressive muscle relaxation, yoga, and meditation can help you relax and manage stress more effectively.

7. **Professional Help:** If stress becomes overwhelming, it may be beneficial to seek help from a mental health professional. They can guide you towards effective coping strategies tailored to your needs.

Strengthening your coping mechanisms is a continual process that can lead to better stress management, improved job satisfaction, and overall greater well-being. Remember, the goal is not to eliminate stress completely—that's often not possible—but to manage it in a way that promotes health and happiness. You can't always control what happens in your work environment, but you can control how you respond. And that can make all the difference.

# 12

# Chapter 12: Building a Supportive Work Environment

The work environment and culture significantly influence the stress levels experienced by employees. A supportive work environment can foster a sense of camaraderie, mutual respect, and understanding that can reduce overall work stress. It can also lead to improved job satisfaction and performance, better patient care, and lower turnover rates. This chapter focuses on strategies to create a work culture that supports and uplifts its members.

### Understanding the Importance of a Supportive Work Environment

A supportive work environment isn't just a nice-to-have; it's a critical component of a healthy workplace. In such environments, employees feel valued, heard, and respected. They're encouraged to express their ideas, share their concerns, and seek help when needed. This leads to lower stress levels, greater job satisfaction, higher levels of creativity and innovation, and better team collaboration.

### Building a Supportive Work Environment

Building a supportive work environment involves actions at different levels, from organizational policies to individual behaviors. Here's how you can contribute:

1. **Promote Open Communication:** Encourage open and honest communication. Make it safe for employees to express their ideas, ask questions, and voice their concerns without fear of retribution.

2. **Foster Collaboration:** Promote a team-based approach to work. Encourage collaboration and the sharing of ideas and knowledge.

3. **Recognize and Value Contributions:** Regularly acknowledge and appreciate employees' efforts. Recognition can go a long way in enhancing motivation and job satisfaction.

4. **Support Work-Life Balance:** Understand that employees have lives outside work. Be supportive of their personal commitments and encourage a healthy work-life balance.

5. **Provide Professional Development Opportunities:** Provide opportunities for employees to learn and grow. This not only enhances their skills but also contributes to their career satisfaction.

6. **Create a Positive Physical Environment:** A clean, well-lit, and comfortable physical environment can reduce stress and improve productivity.

7. **Encourage Peer Support:** Foster an environment where employees support each other during stressful times. This could be through informal chats, peer mentorship programs, or regular team-building activities.

8. **Promote Employee Wellness:** Encourage employees to take care of their physical and mental health. This could be through wellness programs, flexible schedules, or providing resources for self-care and stress management.

Building a supportive work environment is not a one-time task but a continuous effort. It requires the commitment of everyone in the organization—from the top management to the frontline workers. But the benefits are worth it—a supportive work environment not only reduces stress but also leads to happier, healthier, and more productive employees. And ultimately, this leads to better patient care, which is the primary goal of any pharmacy practice.

# 13

# Chapter 13: Navigating Patient Relationships

I n pharmacy practice, building strong relationships with patients is paramount. It not only contributes to effective patient care but also influences a pharmacist's job satisfaction and stress levels. However, managing patient relationships can be challenging—dealing with varying expectations, handling difficult situations, and maintaining professional boundaries. This chapter provides strategies to navigate these complex relationships effectively.

### The Importance of Patient Relationships in Pharmacy

Building strong relationships with patients is essential in pharmacy practice. It improves patient trust and compliance, leads to better health outcomes, and enhances job satisfaction. However, it's important to remember that as a pharmacist, your primary role is to provide professional healthcare advice and services.

### Building Strong Patient Relationships

1. **Empathy and Active Listening:** Show empathy and actively listen to your patients' concerns. This creates a supportive environment where patients feel comfortable sharing their needs.
2. **Clear Communication:** Communicate clearly and in a language that your

patients understand. Avoid medical jargon and ensure they understand their medications and the importance of adherence.

3. **Respect and Dignity:** Treat every patient with respect and dignity, regardless of their background or health condition.

4. **Reliability:** Be consistent and reliable in providing services. This builds patient trust in you and the pharmacy.

5. **Patient Education:** Regularly educate patients about their medications, potential side effects, and any other health-related topics. This not only increases their health literacy but also empowers them to manage their health better.

## Managing Expectations

It's essential to manage patients' expectations to avoid misunderstandings and conflicts. Be transparent about what they can expect from you, including your role, availability, and the services you provide. If their expectations exceed your professional role or capabilities, guide them to the appropriate resources or professionals.

### Dealing with Difficult Situations

Despite your best efforts, difficult situations may arise. These could be due to misunderstandings, unmet expectations, or complex health issues. Here's how to handle them:

1. **Stay Calm and Professional:** Always maintain your composure and professionalism. This can help defuse the situation and keep the conversation focused on finding a solution.

2. **Empathetic Listening:** Allow the patient to express their concerns without interruption. Acknowledge their feelings and concerns, even if you disagree with them.

3. **Resolve Conflicts Constructively:** Aim to resolve conflicts in a way that addresses the patient's concerns while maintaining the boundaries of your professional role.

4. **Seek Support:** If a situation escalates beyond your control, seek support from your colleagues, supervisor, or the pharmacy's protocol for

managing difficult patient situations.

Navigating patient relationships effectively is an art that can be honed with time, patience, and practice. While it may be challenging, remember that these relationships are at the heart of pharmacy practice. They not only allow you to make a positive difference in your patients' health but also enhance your professional satisfaction and reduce work-related stress.

# 14

# Chapter 14: Time Management for Pharmacists

ime management is a critical skill for pharmacists. With the demands of filling prescriptions, counseling patients, administrative tasks, and more, it can often feel like there aren't enough hours in the day. Efficient time management can help balance your workload, reduce feelings of overwhelm, and ensure you have time for relaxation and recuperation. This chapter provides expert advice on how to manage your time effectively.

**Understanding the Value of Time Management in Pharmacy**

Effective time management allows you to be more productive and reduces the potential for errors that can occur when you're rushed. By properly managing your time, you can decrease your stress levels, increase job satisfaction, and improve the quality of care you provide to your patients.

**Time Management Strategies for Pharmacists**

1. **Prioritize Your Tasks:** All tasks are not created equal. Understand which tasks are urgent and important, and prioritize them accordingly. The Eisenhower Matrix is a simple tool that can help you categorize your tasks into four quadrants based on their urgency and importance.

2. **Use a Planner or Digital Calendar:** Keeping track of your tasks and deadlines visually can help ensure nothing slips through the cracks. Use

a planner or digital calendar to organize your schedule.

3. **Delegate Where Possible:** If you have the support of a pharmacy team, delegate tasks appropriately. This can lighten your workload and allows you to focus on tasks that require your specific expertise.

4. **Batch Similar Tasks:** Group similar tasks together to improve efficiency. This could include administrative tasks, patient counseling, or checking prescriptions.

5. **Avoid Multitasking:** Contrary to popular belief, multitasking can reduce productivity and increase the potential for errors. Focus on one task at a time before moving on to the next.

6. **Take Regular Breaks:** Taking short, regular breaks can actually improve your productivity and reduce fatigue. Even a quick five-minute break can help reset your focus and energy levels.

7. **Limit Distractions:** Identify potential distractions in your workplace and find strategies to limit them. This could include setting specific times to check emails, putting your phone on silent, or creating a quiet, focused work environment.

8. **Implement Technology:** Where possible, leverage technology to automate tasks. This can free up your time for more critical, patient-focused duties.

9. **Maintain a Work-Life Balance:** Ensure you set boundaries between your professional and personal life. Remember to allocate time for relaxation and activities you enjoy.

Managing your time effectively is an ongoing process, and different strategies may work better for different people. However, by implementing some of these strategies, you can improve your efficiency, reduce work-related stress, and enhance your professional and personal life.

# 15

# Chapter 15: Managing Career Progression and Expectations

Career progression is a significant part of any professional journey, including pharmacy. Setting realistic career goals, managing expectations, and finding satisfaction in your practice are all essential for long-term success and stress reduction. This chapter provides a guide on how to manage these aspects of your career effectively.

**Setting Realistic Career Goals**

Setting realistic and achievable career goals is the first step towards successful career progression. These goals provide direction, motivation, and a sense of purpose. Follow these steps:

1. **Self-Assessment:** Understand your strengths, weaknesses, interests, and values. This provides a solid foundation for setting career goals that align with your abilities and aspirations.
2. **Research:** Gather information about different career paths in pharmacy. This can include roles in community pharmacies, hospitals, academia, industry, public health, and more.
3. **Set SMART Goals:** Your career goals should be Specific, Measurable, Achievable, Relevant, and Time-bound (SMART). This ensures that your goals are clear, trackable, and within your capabilities.

4. **Create an Action Plan:** Once you have set your goals, create a step-by-step action plan. This should include specific actions, timelines, and resources required to achieve your goals.

**Managing Career Expectations**

Managing career expectations is just as important as setting goals. Unrealistic or unmanaged expectations can lead to dissatisfaction, frustration, and stress. Consider these points:

1. **Understand the Reality of the Profession:** Pharmacy, like any profession, has its challenges. Be prepared for the realities of the job, such as long hours, dealing with difficult patients, or navigating insurance issues.
2. **Be Flexible:** Your career may not always go as planned. Be open to new opportunities and be prepared to adjust your expectations and goals as needed.
3. **Maintain Work-Life Balance:** While career progression is important, it should not come at the expense of your personal life or well-being. Ensure you maintain a balance between work and personal time.

**Finding Satisfaction in Pharmacy Practice**

Career satisfaction contributes to lower stress levels, higher job performance, and overall well-being. Here are some strategies:

1. **Continuous Learning:** Embrace lifelong learning. This can enhance your skills, keep you updated with the latest developments, and provide a sense of achievement.
2. **Mentorship:** Seek mentorship from experienced pharmacists. They can provide guidance, support, and insights from their own career journeys.
3. **Contribute to the Profession:** Participate in professional associations, contribute to research, or mentor younger professionals. This can provide a sense of contribution and satisfaction.
4. **Celebrate Achievements:** Recognize and celebrate your achievements, no matter how small. This can boost your motivation and job satisfaction.

By setting realistic career goals, managing expectations, and finding sat-isfaction in your work, you can navigate your pharmacy career effectively. Remember, everyone's career path is unique, and success is not just about reaching a destination—it's also about enjoying the journey.

# 16

# Chapter 16: Continuing Education without Overwhelm

As a pharmacist, continuing education is not just a requirement for maintaining your license—it's also crucial for staying up-to-date with the latest advancements in the field. However, constant study and exams can add to stress, especially when balanced with a busy work schedule. This chapter offers tips on managing continuing education without feeling overwhelmed.

**Understanding the Importance of Continuing Education**

Continuing education keeps pharmacists abreast of the latest developments in drugs, treatments, and patient care strategies. It ensures the information and advice you provide to patients are based on the most recent evidence. Additionally, it can open new career opportunities and improve job satisfaction by enhancing your competence and confidence.

**Balancing Continuing Education with Work and Personal Life**

1. **Create a Study Schedule:** Rather than studying sporadically, create a consistent study schedule. Allocating specific times for study can make the task more manageable and reduce feelings of overwhelm.
2. **Combine Modes of Learning:** Use a combination of learning methods—online courses, workshops, seminars, webinars, or journal clubs.

This not only provides variety but allows flexibility in fitting learning into your schedule.

3. **Use Work Experience:** Your daily work in the pharmacy is a valuable learning experience. Reflect on your experiences, learn from challenges, and keep track of interesting or unusual cases for future reference.

4. **Quality over Quantity:** Focus on the quality of learning, not just the quantity. Choose continuing education activities that are relevant to your practice, interest, or career goals.

5. **Network with Colleagues:** Colleagues can be a valuable source of learning. Sharing experiences, discussing cases, and seeking advice can enrich your knowledge.

6. **Stay Organized:** Keep a record of your continuing education activities, including certificates, important points learned, and how you've applied this knowledge in practice. This can simplify license renewal and provide a sense of accomplishment.

**Managing Exam Stress**

Exams are often a part of continuing education, and they can be a source of stress. Here are some strategies to manage exam stress:

1. **Start Early:** Starting your exam preparation early gives you ample time to study, review, and revise. Cramming at the last minute often increases stress and can impact performance.

2. **Practice Relaxation Techniques:** Techniques such as deep breathing, mindfulness, or yoga can help reduce stress and improve focus.

3. **Take Care of Your Health:** Regular exercise, a balanced diet, and adequate sleep can improve your energy levels, mood, and cognitive function—boosting your study and exam performance.

4. **Maintain Perspective:** Remember, an exam is just one part of your continuing education and career. Don't let it overshadow the joy of learning and the satisfaction of improving as a professional.

In conclusion, continuing education is a critical component of your career as a pharmacist. By planning, staying organized, and focusing on quality learning, you can manage your continuing education without feeling overwhelmed.

# 17

# Chapter 17: Financial Stress and Pharmacists

Financial stress can significantly impact your well-being and performance at work. As a pharmacist, you may encounter financial stressors like student loan debts, business overheads, or the costs of continual professional development. This chapter offers advice on managing financial stress and planning for a stable and stress-free financial future.

### Understanding Financial Stress

Financial stress occurs when you're unable to meet your financial commitments or when you're constantly worried about your financial situation. This can be caused by factors like high levels of debt, low income, lack of savings, or unexpected expenses. Financial stress can lead to physical health problems, mental health issues like anxiety and depression, and can impact your performance at work.

### Steps to Manage Financial Stress

1. **Assess Your Financial Situation:** The first step to managing financial stress is to have a clear understanding of your financial situation. Calculate your total income, total expenses, debts, and savings. This gives you a clear picture of where you stand financially.

2. **Create a Budget:** Based on your assessment, create a budget that outlines

your income, fixed expenses, variable expenses, and savings. A budget helps you track your spending, identify unnecessary expenses, and allocate funds for saving.

3. **Pay Off Debts:** If you have debts, especially high-interest ones, make a plan to pay them off as soon as possible. You may need to cut back on some expenses or look for additional sources of income. If student loans are a major concern, investigate repayment plans and loan forgiveness programs for healthcare professionals.

4. **Save and Invest:** Aim to save a certain portion of your income regularly. Even small amounts can accumulate over time. Consider speaking with a financial advisor about investment options that can grow your savings.

5. **Plan for Emergencies:** Life is unpredictable, and unexpected expenses can occur. Create an emergency fund to cover at least three to six months' worth of expenses. This can provide a safety net in case of job loss, illness, or other unexpected expenses.

6. **Think Long-Term:** Plan for your long-term financial goals like buying a house, retirement, or your children's education. Long-term financial planning can provide a sense of security and reduce financial stress.

**Stress-Free Financial Future**

1. **Continuous Financial Education:** Stay informed about financial management strategies, investment options, and tax-saving tips. This can help you make informed financial decisions.

2. **Professional Advice:** Consider consulting with a financial advisor. They can provide personalized advice based on your financial situation and goals.

3. **Balance:** While it's important to save and plan for the future, don't forget to enjoy the present. Maintain a balance between spending for the present and saving for the future.

In conclusion, effective financial management can reduce financial stress and contribute to your overall well-being. While it may require discipline and sacrifice, the peace of mind that comes with financial stability is worth the effort.

# 18

# Chapter 18: Seeking Professional Help

Despite best efforts to manage stress in the workplace, there may come a time when professional help is needed. Knowing when to seek such assistance and how to access mental health resources is crucial. This chapter focuses on recognizing the signs of overwhelming stress and provides guidance on how to reach out to professionals for help.

**Recognizing the Need for Help**

Stress is a normal part of life, and everyone experiences it to varying degrees. However, when stress begins to interfere with your ability to function in your personal or professional life, it might be time to seek professional help. Here are some signs that you might need help managing your stress:

1. **Persistent Anxiety or Sadness:** If feelings of anxiety or sadness are affecting your everyday activities and don't seem to improve with time, you might need professional help.
2. **Physical Symptoms:** Stress can manifest as physical symptoms such as headaches, stomach problems, or difficulties with sleep. If these symptoms persist, it's essential to seek help.
3. **Changes in Behavior:** If you notice drastic changes in your behavior, like increased alcohol or drug use, social withdrawal, or loss of interest in activities you once enjoyed, it might indicate the need for professional help.

4. **Impact on Work Performance:** If stress is impacting your work performance, including attention to detail, ability to focus, or interactions with colleagues and patients, it's time to consider professional help.

## Accessing Mental Health Resources

If you feel you need professional help to manage your stress, several resources are available. These include:

1. **Employee Assistance Programs (EAPs):** Many employers offer EAPs that provide services like counseling and referrals for employees experiencing personal or work-related difficulties.
2. **Professional Counseling:** Therapists or counselors can provide techniques to manage stress, treat anxiety or depression, and improve overall mental health.
3. **Psychiatrists:** If necessary, psychiatrists can prescribe medications to help manage symptoms of severe stress, anxiety, or depression.
4. **Support Groups:** Connecting with others who are experiencing similar challenges can provide comfort, reduce feelings of isolation, and provide practical tips.
5. **Online Resources:** Numerous online resources and apps provide stress management techniques, online therapy options, and mental health information.

## Overcoming Barriers to Seeking Help

Many people hesitate to seek help due to stigma, fear, or uncertainty. However, remember that seeking help is a sign of strength, not weakness. It's crucial to prioritize your mental health, and seeking help when needed is an essential part of that.

In conclusion, recognizing when stress becomes too much to handle on your own and seeking professional help is vital. As a pharmacist, taking care of your mental health allows you to provide the best care for your patients and leads to a more fulfilling professional life.

# 19

# Chapter 19: Building a Personal Stress-Reduction Plan

C reating a personalized stress-reduction plan is an essential step towards managing work-related stress. This plan serves as a map to guide you through stress management techniques that cater to your unique needs and challenges. This chapter will provide a step-by-step guide to creating your personal stress-reduction plan.

### Step 1: Identify Your Stressors

The first step in creating a personal stress-reduction plan is identifying your stressors. These could be related to your job, personal life, financial situation, health, or relationships. Write these down in a list format.

### Step 2: Analyze Your Current Coping Strategies

Reflect on how you currently cope with these stressors. Are these strategies healthy or unhealthy? For instance, do you resort to excessive caffeine intake, alcohol, or neglecting your physical health? Not all coping strategies are beneficial, so this step will help you discern which habits to maintain and which to change.

### Step 3: Define Your Stress-Reduction Goals

Define what you want to achieve with your stress-reduction plan. It could be improved mental well-being, increased productivity at work, better relationships, or enhanced physical health. Be as specific as possible with your goals.

### Step 4: Develop New Coping Strategies

Based on your goals, identify new coping strategies that can help you deal with your stressors effectively. Use the knowledge gained from previous chapters to select strategies that are most likely to work for you. These could include mindfulness techniques, physical activities, communication improvements, or changes in work habits.

### Step 5: Plan for Implementation

For each coping strategy, create a specific action plan. When and how will you implement each strategy? How will you overcome potential obstacles? For example, if you plan to start meditating, determine when you'll meditate each day, where you'll do it, and what resources you'll use (like a guided meditation app).

### Step 6: Seek Support

Identify who can support you in your stress-reduction journey. This could be a trusted colleague, family member, friend, or mental health professional. Share your plan with them and ask for their support and accountability.

### Step 7: Review and Adjust Your Plan

A personal stress-reduction plan is not static. It needs to be flexible and adaptable. Regularly review your plan and adjust it based on what's working, what's not, and any changes in your stressors or circumstances.

In conclusion, building a personal stress-reduction plan empowers you to take control of your stress levels. This plan is a dynamic tool that can evolve with your needs and help you manage work-related stress in a proactive and effective way.

# 20

# Chapter 20: Beyond Stress - Towards a Balanced Life

After understanding stress and its management strategies in a professional setting, the journey does not end. Managing stress is just one aspect of fostering a holistic, balanced lifestyle. This chapter will provide final thoughts on integrating all aspects of your life, beyond your pharmacy practice, to achieve overall health and well-being.

### The Importance of a Balanced Lifestyle

Maintaining a balanced lifestyle is crucial for overall health and well-being. A balanced life means that you're giving appropriate time and energy to different areas of your life such as work, relationships, personal interests, health, and relaxation. Having balance helps to ensure that you're not overextending yourself in one area at the expense of others, which can lead to stress and burnout.

### Keys to a Balanced Lifestyle

1. **Work-Life Integration:** Achieving work-life integration means finding a harmony between your professional responsibilities and personal life. This might involve setting boundaries to ensure that work does not encroach on personal time and vice versa.
2. **Physical Health:** Regular exercise, a balanced diet, and adequate sleep

are pillars of physical health. They not only help manage stress but also enhance your energy levels, mood, and overall well-being.

3. **Mental Health:** Prioritize your mental health by practicing mindfulness, seeking professional help when needed, and maintaining a positive mindset. Regularly engaging in activities that you enjoy can also contribute to your mental well-being.

4. **Relationships:** Foster healthy relationships with family, friends, and colleagues. Social support is crucial for stress management and overall happiness.

5. **Personal Development:** Engage in activities that facilitate personal growth and fulfillment. This could include hobbies, learning new skills, or volunteering.

6. **Financial Stability:** As discussed in previous chapters, financial stress can be a significant burden. Achieving financial stability through wise management and planning can contribute to a balanced life.

**Creating Your Balanced Life**

The path to a balanced life is highly personal and may look different for everyone. Here are a few steps to help you create your balanced life:

1. **Reflect:** Consider what a balanced life looks like for you. What are your priorities? What areas of your life need more attention or less?

2. **Plan:** Based on your reflection, create a plan to bring more balance into your life. This might involve adjusting your work schedule, making time for physical activity, or setting financial goals.

3. **Implement:** Put your plan into action. Remember, change often comes gradually. Celebrate small victories and don't be too hard on yourself if progress is slow.

4. **Review:** Regularly review your plan and make adjustments as needed. Your needs and circumstances might change over time, so your plan should be flexible.

In conclusion, stress management is an essential part of a balanced lifestyle, but it doesn't stop there. Integrating all aspects of your life holistically will contribute to your overall health, happiness, and fulfillment, both within and beyond your pharmacy practice.